Cover designed by: Hiremenow
Printed in the United States of America

HOW TO FIGHT OBESITY WITH KETO

Lose Weight Feel Great with Ketogenic Recipes

(For Lazy Keto, Beginners, and Intermediate Low-Carb, High-Fat is Not a Diet But a Lifestyle)

INTRODUCTION

Obesity is a significant health problem in the world today. In fact, according to CDC, approximately 69.2% of Americans over the age of 20 are either overweight or obese! Globally, this translates to 13% of adults living with obesity, according to 2016 statistics.

Worst still, at least 15 percent of school-going children are obese. Sadly, the number of overweight school-age kids and adolescents with obesity has risen more than 10-fold in just under 40 years.

Being obese presents several health problems, such as the increased risk of suffering from certain conditions, mental health problems, and low self-esteem. Thus, it is crucial to address the issue before it is too late.

Probably you have tried different approaches to weight loss, but nothing seems to work. Don't lose hope just yet because this book will introduce you to the ketogenic diet that is quite effective for weight loss.

Various scientific studies have repeatedly shown that a low carb, high fat diet leads to more significant weight loss in overweight children and adults than all other low-fat or low-calorie diets combined. This is what the ketogenic diet is all about, and this book will teach you everything you need to know about this diet to lose weight, achieve your weight loss goals, and feel great.

TABLE OF CONTENTS

AN IN-DEPTH ANALYSIS OF OBESITY

So, what is obesity? When are you considered obese? When obese, you have a body mass index (BMI) of more than 30. BMI is a tool used to assess if someone has the right weight depending on their sex, age, and height. The BMI value is calculated by dividing your weight by the square of your size, converted into meters. A BMI ranging from 25 to 29.9 is considered overweight, while a BMI below 18.5 is considered underweight. Usually, you are deemed to have average weight if your BMI ranges from 18.5 to 24.9, whereas any value beyond 30 is considered "being obese."

Obesity is categorized in various classes depending on its severity. For instance, having a BMI of above 35 is considered **morbid obesit**y, particularly for people weighing 100 pounds over optimal body weight. A body mass index of 35.0-39.9 is referred to as **Class II Obesity**, while above 40 is **exceptionally Obese.**

Any class of obesity is linked to the onset of other life-threatening conditions, diabetes, high blood pressure, arthritis, and some cancer cases. Losing weight through proper diet and exercise and maintaining a healthy weight can significantly help avoid such complications.

Before we move on to the diet part, let us first look at what causes obesity

CAUSES OF OBESITY

Most people assume that obesity is just caused by eating more than your body needs. However, it is much more than this. In this section, we will address the various causes of obesity in addition to eating more calories.

Eating so many calories

Consuming a high amount of calories than your body needs will lead to weight gain, ultimately causing obesity. It is important to note that eating much food does not necessarily lead to weight gain; instead, eating foods high in calories. Below are some of the common culprits:

- Fried foods, among them French fries
- Fatty and processed meats
- Most dairy products
- Fast foods
- High carb foods such as bagels, bread, and other wheat products
- Foods with artificial sugar such as cookies and breakfast cereals
- Artificially sweetened drinks such as sodas and store-bought juices
- Canned and packaged foods with hidden sugars such as ketchup
- High-calorie beverages such as soda, alcohol

In addition, to eating these foods, other poor eating habits such as eating for comfort may lead to obesity.

Sedentary Lifestyle

Lack of physical exercises such as walking, cycling, climbing stairs, or doing a few squats and push-ups contributes to a sedentary lifestyle. You may find yourself working while seated in the office for long hours, then you get home to your TV, and you spend the rest of the evening on your couch. According to a research study, physical activity was found to influence how hormones work, which may indirectly contribute to weight gain. The study suggests that having regular physical activity can help boost various aspects of your health, particularly insulin sensitivity. The type of physical activity and its intensity can affect how your body burns calories, whether in the short and long term.

Lack of enough sleep

I bet you did not expect this, but lack of sleep can make you gain weight. A review study involving 15,000 adults and over 28,000 children suggests that lack of enough sleep directly increases the risk of obesity in adults and children, even those five years old. The researchers discovered that not having enough sleep can lead to obesity since it causes hormonal changes that trigger a high appetite. Lack of sleep triggers the release of the ghrelin hormone (hunger hormone), which significantly boosts appetite while simultaneously suppressing leptin hormone (satiety hormone) that helps curb hunger and unnecessary cravings.

Endocrine disruptors

A 2012 research suggests that liquid fructose, a type of sugar found in sodas, can alter glucose and lipid metabolism and result in health conditions such as fatty liver, cardiovascular disease, high blood pressure, and type II diabetes. High fructose intake is also linked to inflammation, oxidative stress, and other metabolic changes.

Here are few ways to reduce your intake of high fructose and other additives:

- Reduce intake of sodas, sports drinks, and energy drinks

- Eating less coffee creamer, ice cream, and candies

- Avoiding the use of barbecue sauce, ketchup, salad dressings, and other sauces or condiments

- Moderate intake of sweetened foods such as juices, yogurt, and canned foods

- Double-checking nutrition labels to ensure no artificial sugar is added

- Eating unprocessed foods or those unsweetened versions of foods

- Preparing home-based sauces or condiments

When embracing the ketogenic diet, you will remove most of the foods above from your diet.

Genetics

People who suffer from genetic conditions such as Prader-Willi syndrome are more at risk of developing obesity. However, while genetic traits from the parents, such as an enormous appetite, can cause obesity, this doesn't necessarily mean one cannot lose weight by making better lifestyle choices. You may have learned poor eating habits right from childhood, resulting in obesity, rather than just having it in your genes.

Medical reasons

Medical conditions are also to blame for obesity, or at least being overweight. Such medical problems may include:

- Cushing's syndrome, where there's high production of steroid hormones in the body

- Hypothyroidism or an underactive thyroid gland that fails to produce relevant hormones

Often, you can get treatment for most of these health conditions if adequately diagnosed.

Other risk factors for obesity:

- Aging, since it slows down metabolism
- Pregnancy and menopause as a result of hormonal disturbances
- Quitting smoking, which is linked to increased appetite
- Emotional factors such as stress, anxiety, and depression
- A poor economic status, which contributes to poor food choices

I will address some complications of obesity so that you know what is at risk if you do not take the necessary steps to do something now:

COMPLICATIONS OF BEING OBESE

Let's see some of the difficulties:

- Hypertension, or high blood pressure
- High blood cholesterol that blocks arteries leading to heart attack, stroke, and other cardiovascular problems
- Type 2 diabetes
- Cancer, whereas 40% of cancer cases are blamed on obesity
- Kidney disease
- Asthma
- Osteoarthritis since the excess body weight causes strain on bones, joints, and muscles
- Sleep apnea, caused by fat deposits in the neck
- Gastroesophageal reflux. Heartburn and hiatal hernia since the excess weight pushes the valve at the top of the stomach
- Gallbladder disease, since one-point increment BMI increases the risk of this disease by seven percentage points.

As you can see, being obese can result in many life-threatening complications, some that you may have already experienced.

What next now?

The first step is working on your diet. One of the best diets known to help with weight loss is the ketogenic diet.

KETOGENIC DIET FOR OBESITY

In a nutshell, the Ketogenic diet or the Keto diet is a low-carb, high-fat diet aimed at shifting your body's fuel source from default glucose to fats, utilizable in the form of fatty acids and ketones. A low-carb, high fat and moderate protein diet help the body enter **ketosis**, *a process where the body shifts to utilizing fat for fuel.* With lower carbohydrate and protein intake, your body has to burn stored fat to fuel the body. Because fat is an inefficient form of energy (which is why the body prefers carbs), the body has to burn tons of it to provide power for critical bodily functions. Thus, a diet that promotes ketosis can effectively help you shed off extra fat. Because the diet focuses on healthy satiating fats, it effectively lowers cravings and fights occasional hunger.

Before moving forward, let us look at why eating carbohydrates mainly leads to weight gain

When you eat a meal rich in carbohydrates, the body breaks down carbs into glucose in the digestive tract for fuel. Glucose is generally preferred for power. It offers your body cells the most reliable source of ATP, the primary source of energy molecule required to facilitate all bodily processes. After digestion, the glucose is absorbed into the bloodstream, where it temporarily causes a spike in blood glucose level. Your body then produces insulin hormone that facilitates glucose uptake into body cells and regulates blood sugar levels.

While all this sounds okay, having high blood sugar levels frequently due to continuous intake of high-carb food is problematic. So what then does the body do with all the glucose in the bloodstream? Insulin helps the body cells to take up the glucose; thus, lowering blood sugar levels. For the excess, your body has various mechanisms of saving up energy that it doesn't need at the moment, which include:

GLYCOGENESIS

This is the process where any excess glucose is further converted into glycogen for storage in body areas such as the liver and muscles. According to various researchers, it has been established that the body's storage space for liver and muscle glycogen is a maximum of 2000 calories. Based on your activity level, your glycogen stores will be depleted within 6 to 24 hours when you don't eat any other calories. Most of us hardly go 5 hours before snacking especially high-carb foods; therefore, glycogen stores get filled up, and thereby, another process referred to as lipogenesis is initiated.

LIPOGENESIS

With this process, any extra glycogen in the liver and muscles is converted to fat for a "permanent backup" utilizable beyond 24 hours of fasting. As opposed to limited glycogen stores, bodily fat has a total storage area in your abdomen and other regions. For instance, the visceral fat on the stomach can sustain metabolic processes for several weeks where you hardly eat any food! But as you know, most of us eat at least three meals a day with unhealthy snacking, which ultimately leads to weight gain. The thing with visceral fat is that in addition to causing weight gain, it also increases the risk of suffering from various metabolic disorders such as obesity and heart disease.

As you can see, all these problems begin with extra glucose in the body, obviously from the intake of carbs. When you moderate your carbs intake, both glycogenesis and lipogenesis processes stop. No excess glucose is available. Once your body is starved of glucose, any stored glycogen is converted into glucose through a process called glycogenolysis. If you do not eat carbs, the body is forced to look for alternative energy sources. Here the body is forced to undergo a metabolic process in which the liver begins to synthesize stored fats and fatty acids as a source of fuel. This induced metabolic state where the body is forced to break down stored fats for energy is called *ketosis*. The end product of ketosis is called ketones, which are as effective as glucose in fuelling bodily processes.

The ketogenic diet encourages reducing the consumption of carbohydrates while increasing your intake of fat. You may probably be wondering, wouldn't fat make you fat? First, it is essential to understand that weight loss has a lot to do with insulin level. If your insulin level is high, there is no way you will lose weight and vice versa.

It is critical to understand that dietary fats don't significantly affect blood sugar or insulin levels. Digested glucose from carbohydrates elevates blood sugar level, which triggers the release of insulin hormone. This hormone stimulates cells to "open up" and take in glucose into body cells to fuel various metabolic processes. While insulin is necessary, its secretion into the blood inhibits fat metabolism as the body switches to glucose metabolism for energy. In such scenarios, stored body fat is left intact, which hinders effective fat breakdown, which is a massive blow to weight loss. The Keto diet helps deplete the body of its glucose supply, forcing the body to break down stored fats for energy.

As already stated, protein intake should be moderated to around 20 percent, and for a reason. This is because proteins can affect blood sugar and insulin levels too. Any extra protein in the bloodstream is converted into glucose in what is called *gluconeogenesis*. This translates to an increase in blood sugar, which triggers a rise in insulin levels. As an increase in insulin facilitates glucose metabolism, it directly hinders fat breakdown and overall fat loss. Therefore, to avoid converting protein to glucose, limit intake to about 1-1.5 grams per kilo of lean body mass. With low carb and moderate protein intake, liver glycogen (stored glucose) levels are depleted, making the body break down fatty acids into ketones.

Recently, the Ketogenic diet has become famous for weight loss, treating diabetes, and other metabolic disorders, which has led to many misconceptions about the ketogenic diet. Let us bust a few myths about the ketogenic diet to separate the real from the myths.

BUSTING MYTHS SURROUNDING THE KETOGENIC DIET

In this chapter, we will look at some myths about the ketogenic diet. I will then provide accurate and honest information about the diet to help you understand what you are getting yourself into by adopting the ketogenic diet. Let us get started:

Eating fat causes obesity

Let's face it: some concerns about embracing a high-fat diet triggers obesity in some dieters. While such claims sound reasonable, nothing could be further from the truth! Eating a high-fat diet does not necessarily cause obesity, but rather it's the insulin cycle stimulated by eating high-carb foods that is the culprit. Once you eat a high carb meal, insulin level spikes to facilitate glucose uptake in cells; and rapid absorption of glucose often triggers craving and hunger. Also, high-fat diets, promote satiety and you do not experience the energy lows that come with eating high-carb foods, leading to increased appetite and cravings.

It is also vital to note that not all fat is good; therefore, you should eat more unsaturated fats like avocados, nuts, seeds, olive oil, etc., and not as many saturated fats.

Saturated fat causes heart disease

Some people believe that increasing your intake of saturated fats can raise cholesterol levels and trigger cardiovascular problems.

However, most studies conclude that its increased blood sugar and insulin levels are inflammatory to body cells rather than saturated fats. A research study has found that the Keto diet reduces inflammation linked to heart disease as it is high in saturated fats but low in carbs. The study further states that saturated fats shouldn't directly be responsible for elevated cholesterol levels. Related research found that saturated fats boost "good cholesterol" while reducing dangerous cholesterol (or triglyceride levels). In so doing, the Keto diet reduces the risk of heart disease.

You can eat as much fat as you want on the ketogenic diet

Yes, the ketogenic diet is high in fat, and I have mentioned that fat does not affect insulin levels. However, it is essential to note that the ketogenic diet does not give you the green light to have all kinds of fat. The best way to increase your fat intake is to take more unsaturated fats such as flaxseed, olive oil, avocados, and less saturated fats such as sausage and bacon, not the healthiest.

Calories are not as crucial for weight loss

The keto diet is not a diet that requires you to keep a count of every calorie you eat. However, it is also not an "eat as much as you desire" kind of diet. You cannot wholly forego calories if you desire to lose weight. Yes, you will lose weight in the beginning when you get rid of most of the carbs. However, you still need to be aware of your calorie intake; though, you don't have to be obsessed about it.

Let us now look at how you stand to benefit by getting started on the ketogenic diet:

BENEFITS OF THE KETOGENIC DIET

Here are the benefits you get from adopting the diet:

Weight Loss

The Keto diet can help you burn fat and lose pounds within a few weeks. A research study has shown that when an equal number of calories consumed across different diet plans, a low-carb diet facilitates more significant fat loss. In the study, scientists compared three specific meal plans that contained varying amounts of carbs, i.e., 104, 60, and 30 grams of carbs. They discovered a negative correlation between carbs consumed and weight loss but positively correlated with lean weight loss. A low-carb diet (30 grams) proved to be more effective in losing weight and conserving muscle mass.

Another research found that around 10 grams of carbs were consumed for ten days, participants could lose 97 percent of their total body fat. The study concluded that a low-carb diet is very effective even in obese people and doesn't require dieters to restrict calorie intake too much to lose weight.

A related study corroborated that eating high amounts of fats and protein is more effective in weight loss than a low-fat diet. Another research concluded that obese people with metabolic syndrome or diabetes could lose more weight on Keto than a low-fat diet within a six months time-frame. The study showed that the keto diet could help diabetic people boost their insulin hormone sensitivity and lower triglyceride levels.

In summary, studies have shown that the keto diet is more effective for weight loss than conventional diets, particularly for the first six months. Outcome after six months depends on adherence to the diet but still scores better than other diets. But with strong willpower to achieve proper adherence to the Keto diet, you can lose weight and maintain it within a longer time frame.

Lower blood sugar levels

High blood sugar level, no doubt, is a risk factor for obesity. But how does it get here? To begin with, understand that carbs are broken down into glucose which enters the bloodstream and raises your blood sugar levels. An increase in blood glucose leads to the secretion of *insulin hormone*. The hormone causes blood glucose transported into the cells, and the glucose is stored in the form of glycogen for future use. A high-carb diet will trigger a spike in insulin if you're healthy but may not cause serious problems apart from poor fat metabolism.

But in some dieters, it can seriously affect them. For instance, you can develop insulin resistance which means that your cells cannot absorb the glucose; thus, they cannot control blood glucose levels. If diabetic, your body can fail to produce enough insulin to regulate blood sugar levels in the bloodstream. Medical reports show that having elevated blood glucose can, in the long term, cause weight gain, extreme fatigue, among other problems. Cutting down on the number of carbs can eliminate the need for insulin hormone and related insulin resistance.

With the ketogenic diet, patients on diabetic treatment can lower their dosage by 50 percent without developing complications. Several studies have shown that most diabetics can decrease or eliminate the need for insulin medication within six months of the Keto diet. However, you may need to talk to your physician before reducing your carb intake since abrupt carb withdrawal can cause hypoglycemia, a condition characterized by extremely low blood sugar.

Curbs Hunger and Cravings

The ketogenic diet promotes satiety or fullness, and in-so-doing suppresses hunger and unnecessary cravings that cause you to snack on processed or high-carb foods. One group of obese dieters was put on a 30 percent protein diet and 4 percent carbs in a particular study, while the other group fed 35 percent carbs. Then their body weight and level of ketosis were evaluated using their urine samples and analysis of blood plasma. A computerized system was used to assess and analyze their hunger patterns within four weeks.

After the elapse of 4 weeks, dieters who consumed a 4 percent carb diet had lower consumption of energy and reduced hunger than those who ate 35 percent of carbs. This study concluded that a low-carb and moderate protein diet could help reduce hunger and food intake on a short-term basis. Related research found that obese and non-diabetic overweight dieters can effectively reduce their appetite and lose 13 percent of body weight.

Keeps cholesterol levels in check

You may have heard that high cholesterol is dangerous, but perhaps you don't know that there are two types of cholesterol! We usually have the "good" cholesterol or High-Density Lipoprotein (HDL), and the "bad" cholesterol is referred to as Lower Density Lipoprotein (LDL). The "good" HDL cholesterol comes from healthy fats such as fish oil and avocado, while the LDL comes from saturated fats, particularly those solid at room temperature. Solid fats such as vegetable shortening and stick margarine, fried foods, and most commercially-baked goods contain saturated fats, leading to higher LDL cholesterol levels.

Two types of cholesterol play opposite roles. For instance, HDL helps transport cholesterol away from your body and the liver, which can then be excreted or recycled. But LDL carries the cholesterol from your liver back into body tissues, where it is reabsorbed. Bear in mind that Low-density lipoprotein is attributed to the clogging of the arteries and can inhibit blood flow and oxygen supply to major body organs such as the heart. That said, how does high cholesterol result in cardiovascular problems like heart disease or heart attack?

The buildup of cholesterol in the blood clogs up the arteries in what is referred to as atherosclerosis. The arteries are then narrowed to the extent that blood flow to the heart muscle is blocked. As the blood towards the heart brings fresh oxygen, lack of enough blood or oxygen causes complications such as severe chest pains. However, if blood flow to a portion of your heart is completely blocked off, you might get a heart attack.

One of the best ways to improve cardiovascular health is to eat healthy fats that the ketogenic diet is high. These include foods such as avocado, fish oil, and nuts. These food ingredients contain healthy omega-three fatty acids, which boost "good" cholesterol levels. Based on research, people with higher levels of HDL are less likely to develop cardiovascular problems like the heart disease

I believe having learned the different benefits of the ketogenic diet, you are excited to get started. Let us now look at the foods you will eat:

Let's briefly discuss that.

THE FOODS

As mentioned earlier, the ketogenic diet is a low-carb diet; therefore, you have to reduce the number of carbohydrates consumed significantly. The bulk of the Ketogenic diet is fats and oils and moderate protein intake. We will start by looking at the foods that you will eat

1. FATS AND OILS

The most recommended fats to consume are omega-three fatty oils, including fish like salmon, tuna, and trout, to mention a few. Additionally, you should eat more monounsaturated fats like avocados and coconut oils. These fats are preferred because they have a stable chemical structure, which is less inflammatory. Below is a comprehensive list of great sources of fats you can eat:

- Mozzarella cheese
- Olive oil
- Butter
- Cheddar cheese
- Heavy whipping cream
- Sour cream
- Vegetable oil
- Parmesan cheese
- Organic coconut oil
- Cottage cheese

2. PROTEINS

This food group forms an essential part of the Keto diet plan as it facilitates general growth and repair of worn-out cells. Protein also helps in the synthesis and monitoring of hormones in the bloodstream that control various bodily functions.

Here are examples of meats, fish, poultry, and other protein foods that you can consume:

- Bacon
- Fish such as catfish, trout, salmon, mackerel, tuna, and codfish
- Eggs
- Chorizo
- Duck
- Lamb
- Pork
- Chicken breasts
- Lobster
- Haddock
- Scallops
- Deveined shrimp
- Ham
- Pork sausage rinds

- Ground turkey
- Hot Italian sausage
- Ducks breast
- Turkey pepperoni
- Lean deli ham
- Canned tuna

3. VEGGIES

These are a source of vitamins that enhance your immune system to fight diseases, especially leafy green veggies. It is essential to avoid starchy carbs strictly. Also, try the following veggies, among others:

- Red/Green bell pepper
- Tomatoes
- Onion
- Button mushrooms
- Flat-leaf parsley
- Head leaf lettuce
- Spinach
- Jalapeno pepper
- Zucchini
- Eggplant
- Cauliflower

4. NUTS, SEEDS, AND FRUITS

You can also eat moderate amounts of low-carb fruits, nuts, and seeds to help control carb intake. Here's what to put on your plate:

- Pecans
- Sesame seeds
- Tahini
- Walnuts
- Almond flour
- Flaxseed meal
- Raisins
- Sunflower seeds

Fruits

Most fruits are rich in sugars, fructose, and carbs, and thus you can only eat a few types of them and moderation. You can enjoy:

- Blueberries
- Cranberries
- Avocado
- Strawberries
- Olives

- Coconut
- Blackberries
- Raspberries

5. BEVERAGES/DRINKS

You can enjoy a few drinks but ensure that they are plain or un-sweetened to monitor carb intake.

- Water
- Lemon and lime juice
- Herbal tea
- Almond milk
- Clear broth, bone broth
- Flavored seltzer water
- Decaf tea
- Decaf coffee
- Coconut milk

FOODS TO AVOID

1. SUGARS

Snack foods such as chips, pastries, cookies, pretzels, and wheat thins are your number one enemy since they are processed and contain added sugars. The rule of the thumb is to avoid a majority of sweet products or any food substance that contains sugar, honey, or sucrose. The following are the culprits in terms of high sugar content:

- Brown sugar
- Canned soups and stews
- Fruit juices, fruit syrup, and concentrates
- Rice and maple syrup
- Maltose, barley malt, and malt powder
- Fructose
- Coconut sugar
- Brown rice syrup
- Agave nectar and honey
- Cane sugar, syrup, and cane juice

2. GRAINS AND RELATED PRODUCTS

Avoid all grains and their products such as:

- Pretzels
- Cakes, pies
- Cookies, tarts
- Crackers
- Tortillas
- Cold cereals, hot cereals
- Pasta
- Waffles, pancakes
- Cereals
- Sandwiches
- English muffins
- Wheat Thins
- Bread, muffins, rolls, bread crumbs
- Corn
- High-fructose corn syrup
- Oatmeal
- Whole wheat Pancakes

Ensure that you read the list of ingredients first before you purchase packaged food products.

3. SUGARY BEVERAGES

Most energy drinks, beers, fruit juices, and non-diet sodas are of high sugar and often disrupt fat metabolism as they raise insulin levels. Therefore avoid high-carb beverages among them:

- Alcohol
- Fruits juices
- Sweet or dessert wines
- Non-diet sodas
- Energy drinks

4. STARCHY VEGGIES, TUBERS, AND LEGUMES

Veggies are low-carb, but you should avoid the starchy ones as these don't promote fullness or satiety. These starchy foods include:

- Potatoes
- Lentils
- Yam
- Chickpea
- potato chips
- Artichokes
- Butternut squash
- French fries
- Black-eyed peas
- Soybeans and related products
- Legumes such as green, white, or black beans
- Beets
- Tofu

5. MILK

You should avoid cow milk due to the presence of lactose. Instead, drink yogurt or other fermented milk products. Alternatively, you can drink milk or dairy alternatives such as almond milk, coconut milk, etc. Kindly refer to the allowed beverages on the ketogenic diet.

6. LEGUMES

Though legumes contain a significant quantity of proteins, you should avoid them due to their high starch content. As ketogenic is a low-carb diet, you shouldn't eat any beans, peas, peanuts, and lentils.

To make the transition to the Ketogenic diet as smooth as possible, it's essential to make a meal plan. With a good plan, it's an easy task to consume only ketogenic ingredients of your choice strictly. Here you get ideas on how to get started for the first few days of your diet. These meal ideas can be tweaked with other meals suggested in the grocery list to make your diet flexible.

Consider the following low carb recipes:

KETO-FRIENDLY RECIPES

BREAKFAST

Breakfast Casserole with Sausage

Serves 10

Prep Time: 15 minutes

Cook Time: 35 minutes

Total Time: 50 minutes

Nutritional Information Per Serving: Calories 276, Carbs 5.2g, Protein 17.9g, Fat 20.7g

Ingredients

1/8 teaspoon pepper

1/4 teaspoon sea salt

1/2 cup almond or coconut milk

12 eggs

12 ounces broccoli, chopped

3 cups yellow summer squash cubed

2 cloves garlic, minced

1 pound sausage or other ground meat, nitrate-free

1 tablespoon olive or avocado oil

1/2 teaspoon dry minced onion flakes, optional

Cheese for serving

Directions

1. Begin by cooking the garlic, sausage, and onion flakes, if using, over medium-high heat until the sausage or the ground meat is browned.

2. Add in broccoli and the squash, and then pour into a casserole dish measuring 9x13 inches.

3. Whisk together coconut or almond milk and eggs in a medium bowl, and add pepper and salt.

4. Pour the mixture over the browned sausage. Bake until the eggs are set, and the top begins to brown. This should take you approximately 30 to 35 minutes.

CINNAMON WALNUT MUFFINS

Yields 12 muffins

Prep Time: 10 minutes

Cook Time: 20 minutes

Total Time: 30 minutes

Nutritional information: Calories 219, Carbs 6g, Protein 6g, Fat 20g

Ingredients

1/2 teaspoon baking soda

1 teaspoon lemon juice

2 teaspoons cinnamon

2 teaspoons vanilla extract

1/4 cup coconut flour

1/2 cup erythritol or sugar alcohol sweetener

1/2 cup avocado oil or any oil

4 pastured eggs

1 cup golden flaxseed or flax meal, ground

1 cup walnuts chopped, optional

Pinch of sea salt

Directions

1. Bring your oven to heat at 325 degrees F.

2. Then, grind the flax seeds with a coffee grinder and then measure approximately 1 cup.

3. In a mixing bowl, combine all the ingredients until incorporated or use an electric mixer. Add in walnuts last.

4. Bake the mixture in the preheated oven for approximately 18 to 22 minutes. Consider using muffin liners to prevent any sticking.

KETO SPINACH OMELET

Yields 1 omelet

Prep Time: 10 minutes

Cook Time: 10 minutes

Total Time: 20 minutes

Nutritional information: Calories 266.3, Carbs 11.3g, Protein 29.6g, Fat 9.1g

Ingredients

5 egg whites

1 large egg

1-ounce mozzarella cheese

2 cups organic baby spinach

4 onions, sliced

Directions

1. Heat a pan or skillet.

2. Mix the 5 egg whites with 1 egg and then pour into the pan. Cook until set on one side.

3. Flip over the egg mixture; add the onions, cheese, and spinach on the top, and fold.

5. Serve and enjoy the omelet.

EGGS BENEDICT

Serves 4

Prep Time: 10 minutes

Cook Time: 5 minutes

Total Time: 15 minutes

Nutritional information per serving: Calories 252, Carbs 2g, Protein 15g, Fat 20g

Ingredients

4 halves keto muffins toasted, or sliced tomato

1 batch Keto hollandaise sauce

4 slices Canadian bacon or sliced ham, cooked

4 large eggs

Directions

1. Put 2 to 3 inches of water in a saucepan or deep skillet along with a drop of vinegar.

2. Bring the water to a gentle boil and then lower the heat. Break the eggs slowly into the hot water and cook until the egg whites become firm.

3. Remove the eggs from water using a slotted spoon.

4. Put the slices of tomato or the low carb muffins on plates and top each dish with ham or Canadian bacon.

5. Put the poached eggs on top, and then pour the sauce over

the cooked eggs. Sprinkle with some paprika if you like.

45

CREAM CHEESE PANCAKES

Serves 7

Prep Time: 2 minutes

Cook Time: 7 minutes

Total Time: 9 minutes

Nutritional Information Per Serving: Calories 149, Carbs 1.8g, Protein 7.2g, Fat 12.7g

Ingredients

1 tablespoon whole psyllium husks

15 drops vanilla stevia drops

6 ounces cream cheese

6 large eggs

Directions

1. Put everything in a small food processor or blender and puree until well incorporated.

2. Pour approximately 3 tablespoons of the mixture into a hot frying pan or griddle for each pancake.

3. Cook until the top of the pancake is covered in bubbles and the edges are dry, and then flip.

4. Cook until the bottom side has browned, and then remove the pancake from the skillet.

5. Serve the pancakes warm with some butter and Keto-

friendly maple-flavored syrup if you like.

CHARD & SAUSAGE HASH

Serves 2-4

Total Time: 30 minutes

Nutritional Information Per Serving: Calories 576, Carbs 12.8g, Protein 29.4g, Fat 46g

Ingredients

1 teaspoon Dijon mustard

1 tablespoon fresh lemon juice

2 cloves garlic

3 tablespoons ghee or lard

150g sausage meat, gluten-free

2 cups cauli-rice

200g Swiss chard or dark-leaf kale

Pepper

Salt

4 poached eggs, optional

Directions

1. Rice the cauliflower and set it aside. Cut the stalks from the chard and chop them into tiny pieces.

2. In a large pan greased with some ghee, cook the sausage until it's browned on its sides. Use a slotted spoon to remove it from heat and put it in a bowl.

3. Add ghee to the pan, then peel and finely chop garlic. Put it in the pan and cook until fragrant.

4. Add the cauli-rice and cook for about 5 minutes on medium heat, making sure that you stir occasionally.

5. Then add the mustard, chard stalks, and lemon juice, and cook for 2 minutes. Season the mixture with pepper and salt, and mix well to incorporate.

6. Chop the chard leaves, add to the pan, and cook for 2 minutes. Then add cooked sausage, mix and remove from heat.

7. Top with fried or poached eggs if you like.

CHEESE OMELET

Serves 2

Total Time: 15 minutes

Nutritional Information: Calories 895, Carbs 7g, Proteins 51g, Fat 97g

Ingredients

7 ounces shredded cheddar cheese

6 eggs

3 ounces butter

Salt and pepper to taste

Directions

1. Whisk the eggs until smooth and frothy.

2. Add in half the cheese, season with salt and pepper, and mix.

3. In a hot frying pan, melt some butter and pour in the cheese and egg mixture. Let the contents settle for a couple of minutes.

4. Reduce the heat and then cook until the mixture is well cooked.

5. Add in the rest of the cheese and fold. Serve while hot.

SPINACH AND MOZZARELLA FRITTATA

Serves 3

Prep Time: 15 minutes

Cook Time: 90 minutes

Total Time: 1 hour 15 minutes

Nutritional Information Per Serving: Calories: 127, Carbs 3g, Protein 9g, Fat 9g

Ingredients

1 Roma tomato, diced

Salt to taste

1 cup chopped baby spinach, without stems

1/4 teaspoon white pepper

1/4 teaspoon black pepper

2 tablespoons full-fat milk

3 egg whites

3 eggs

1 cup shredded mozzarella cheese, divided

1/2 cup diced onion

1 tablespoon extra-virgin olive oil

Directions

1. Add oil to a small skillet and sauté the onion for around 5 minutes. Once tender, remove from the skillet and set aside.

2. Using non-stick cooking spray, coat a slow cooker and set it aside.

3. Mix ¾ cup of the cheese, sautéed onion, and the rest of the ingredients. Once mixed, transfer to the Crockpot.

4. Now sprinkle the remaining mozzarella on top of the mixture. Cook the contents on low for 1 hour to 1 ½ hour while covered.

5. As soon as the eggs are set, remove them from the cooker and serve.

FLUFFY KETO WAFFLE

Serves 4

Prep Time: 10 minutes

Cook Time: 15 minutes

Total Time: 25 minutes

Nutritional Information Per Serving: Calories 200, Carbs 5g, Protein 9g, Fat 15g

Ingredients

Batter:

1/2 teaspoon maple extract

1 dash cinnamon

1 1/2 teaspoons baking powder

4 tablespoons coconut flour

1 tablespoon sugar substitute

2 teaspoons vanilla extract, sugar-free

4 eggs

4 ounces cream cheese, softened

Almond milk as needed

Directions

1. To make the waffles, mix eggs, cinnamon, sugar substitute, maple extract, vanilla, and cream cheese using a mixer or blender.

2. Then add in melted butter along with coconut flour and baking powder. Blend the mixture until fully incorporated.

3. If the batter thickens after a few minutes, add a splash of almond milk, half and half, and cream to make it thinner.

4. Pour the batter into a preheated iron and cook until golden brown or for about 5 to 7 minutes.

5. Serve the waffles with sugar-free syrup or butter.

MEXICAN BREAKFAST CASSEROLE

Serves 10

Prep Time: 15 minutes

Cook Time: 2 hours 30 minutes

Total Time: 2 hours 45 minutes

Nutritional Information Per Serving: Calories 284, Carbs 3g, Protein 15g, Fat 23g

Ingredients

1 cup Pepper Jack cheese

1 cup almond milk

10 eggs

1 cup salsa

1/4 teaspoon pepper

1/4 teaspoon salt

1 teaspoon chili powder

1 teaspoon cumin

1/2 teaspoon coriander

1/2 teaspoon garlic powder

12 ounces Pork Sausage Roll

Avocado salsa, sour cream, cilantro- optional

Directions

1. First, cook the pork sausage in a large skillet over medium heat until it's no longer pink.

2. Season and add salsa, then set aside to cool down slightly.

3. In a separate bowl, whisk the coconut milk with eggs, then add pork to the eggs.

4. Now add in Jack cheese and stir to mix. Grease the bottom of a slow cooker and pour in the egg mixture.

5. Finally, cook on low for 5 hours or high for 2 ½ hours. Serve topped with preferred toppings.

SALADS

BASIL SPINACH SALAD

Serves 2

Total Time: 15 minutes

Nutritional Information Per Serving: Calories 146, Carbs 15g, Protein 5g, Fat 7g

Ingredients

½ cup basil, fresh, several sprigs

4 cups spinach

2 medium tomatoes, diced

½ medium onions, yellow, diced

1 tablespoon coconut oil

Directions

1. Begin by washing and preparing the veggies.

2. Heat a small skillet over medium heat, and add in coconut oil when fully hot.

3. Now add in diced onions, and sauté the mixture until soft and translucent. Now add in the tomatoes and then cook for 2 more minutes.

4. Finally, add basil and spinach to the pan, cook for 1 more minute, and then serve it warm.

KETO SARDINE SALAD

Serves 1

Prep Time: 5 minutes

Cook Time: 0 minutes

Total Time: 5 minutes

Nutritional Information Per Serving: Calories 400, Carbs 2g, Protein 30g, Fat 34g

Ingredients

1 tablespoon lemon juice

1 tablespoon olive oil

1/10 pounds bacon or leftover meat, chopped small

1/4 pound salad greens

1 (4-ounce) can sardine in olive oil or brine, drained

Salt to taste

Directions

1. Toss the salad greens in lemon juice and olive oil. Add in the bacon or leftover meat and toss to combine.

2. Toss the mixture with drained fish and sprinkle with salt.

3. Serve and enjoy.

CHEESE & SPINACH SALAD BOWL

Serves 2

Total Time: 25 minutes

Nutritional Information Per Serving: Calories 645, Carbs 9.8 g, Protein 33.2g, Fat 54.2g

Ingredients

½ cup flaked almonds, toasted

4 cups fresh spinach

1 ½ cups hard goat cheese, grated

4 strawberries for garnish

Directions

1. Preheat the oven to 400 degrees F. Use parchment paper- cut in half to line a baking tray.

2. Grate the goat cheese onto the baking sheet in the shape of two rough circles.

3. Place the cheese in the preheated oven and bake for 10 minutes. Once golden in color, remove from the oven and cool down.

4. Place a small bowl upside down, and then lift the parchment paper off the tray. Now flip the cheese over the bowl. Press the edges lightly and allow to cool for about 5 minutes.

5. Make salad filling, pat-dry-washed spinach with a paper towel, and put it in the cheese bowls.

6. Toss with salad filling, and sprinkle with almond flakes, toasted. If desired, top with strawberry slices.

KETO TUNA SALAD

Serves 1

Total Time: 5 minutes

Nutritional Information Per Serving: Calories 626, Carbs 5.4g, Protein 41.4g, Fat 49.7g

Ingredients

1 tablespoon extra virgin olive oil

1 tablespoon lemon juice, fresh

1 medium spring onion or a bunch of chives

2 tablespoon mayonnaise

2 eggs, hard-boiled

140g tinned tuna, drained

1 small head of lettuce

Pink Himalayan salt

Directions

1. Tear the leaves from lettuce, wash and pat dry using a paper towel or drain in a salad spinner.

2. Spread the leaves at the bottom of a salad bowl. Add drained and shredded fish.

3. Top the tuna with hard-boiled eggs, chopped spring onion, and mayo. If desired, drizzle with olive oil.

CAESAR SALAD

Serves 4

Prep Time: 15 minutes

Cook Time: 12 minutes

Total Time: 27 minutes

Nutritional Information Per Serving: Calories 269, Carbs 13g, Protein 31g, Fat 10g

Ingredients

1 1/4 cups croutons, fat-free

8 cups romaine lettuce, cut into 2-inch strips

1/4 cup shaved fresh parmesan cheese,

2 tablespoons grated parmesan cheese

1 tablespoon water

1/2 teaspoon anchovy paste

3/4 teaspoon minced garlic

1 teaspoon Worcestershire sauce

1 1/2 teaspoons red wine vinegar

1 1/2 teaspoons Dijon mustard

1 tablespoon extra-virgin olive oil

2 tablespoons fresh lemon juice

1/2 cup silken soft tofu

1/4 and 1/8 teaspoon black pepper, freshly ground

1/4 and 1/8 teaspoon kosher salt, divided

1 pound chicken skinless and boneless breast halves

Olive oil cooking spray

Directions

1. Heat a grill pan to medium heat.

2. Meanwhile, coat the chicken breasts using olive oil spray. Season the misted meat breast with a ¼ teaspoon of pepper and salt.

3. Grill your chicken until it's cooked through, or for about 5-6 minutes per side.

4. Cool the cooked chicken on a cutting board for about 5 minutes to help distribute juices. When cool, cut your chicken into bite-size pieces.

5. Into a blender, combine the soft tofu, minced garlic, fresh lemon juice, red wine vinegar, extra-virgin olive oil, Dijon mustard, Worcestershire sauce, anchovy paste, and then add the remaining pepper and salt.

6. Process the ingredients until thoroughly combined and creamy. If necessary, scrape down the blender sides. To thin the creamy mixture, you can add about a tablespoon of water. Now stir in the grated Parmesan.

7. In a large bowl, toss the dressing, lettuce, and croutons, and then divide the mixture into four serving plates.

8. At this point, put the chicken over the salad and then sprinkle shaved Parmesan onto each plate.

MUSHROOM SALAD

Serves 2

Prep Time: 5 minutes

Cook Time: 10 minutes

Total Time: 15 minutes

Nutritional Information Per Serving: Calories 117, Carbs 11g, Protein 5.6g, Fat 7.5g

Ingredients

1-2 tablespoons lemon juice

A pinch of black pepper

½ teaspoon sea salt

1 tablespoon coconut oil or olive oil

Zest of ½ lemon

2 garlic cloves, peeled and diced

5 springs of fresh thyme, leaves only

10-11 ounces sliced button mushrooms

Cracked black pepper, to taste

Directions

1. In a large frying pan, heat some the until hot, and then add in the mushrooms.

2. Cook on high until browned or for about 3 to 4 minutes, and then lower the heat to medium.

3. Flip the mushrooms over as soon as they start to release a liquid. Cook the other side for around 2 minutes.

4. Now add in thyme, garlic, pepper, butter, lemon zest, and sea salt, and cook for about 1-2 minutes while stirring.

4. At this point, drizzle with some fresh lemon juice, toss a little to incorporate together, and then serve.

ARTICHOKE AND ASPARAGUS SALAD

Serves 2-3

Prep Time: 10 minutes

Cook Time: 5 minutes

Total Time: 15 minutes

Nutritional Information Per Serving: Calories 184, Carbs 12g, Protein 11g, Fats 10g

Ingredients

1 ounce shaved Parmesan cheese

1 pound medium asparagus, cut into thirds

1 (14-ounce) can of artichoke hearts, quartered

1/4 teaspoon pepper

1/4 teaspoon salt

1/2 teaspoon dried oregano

1 tablespoon lemon juice, fresh

2 tablespoons extra-virgin olive oil

1 garlic clove, peeled and halved lengthwise

Directions

1. Rub the insides of a salad bowl with garlic clove. Throw away the garlic.

2. Then add pepper, salt, oregano, lemon juice, and oil. Whisk the contents entirely and then add in artichokes.

3. Toss the mixture slowly and allow to rest for some time at average room temperature.

4. Put the asparagus in salted boiling water, and cook until crisp-tender.

5. When crisp-tender, rinse under cool water, drain and then blot dry using a paper towel.

6. Add the asparagus into the artichoke mixture, and then well.

7. Serve the salad, then sprinkle the shaved Parmesan over each salad bowl and serve.

BACON & ASPARAGUS SALAD

Serves 2

Prep Time: 20 minutes

Total Time: 30 minutes

Ingredients

Nutritional Information Per Serving: Calories 216, Carbs 6g, Protein 9.5g, Fat 18g

For the Dressing:

1/2 teaspoon mixed herbs: dill, chervil, or tarragon

1/4 teaspoon pepper

1/2 teaspoon salt

1 lemon, juiced

1 tablespoon Dijon mustard

1/4 cup olive oil

For the Salad:

1 shallot, finely sliced, sautéed until crisp in oil

1 avocado, sliced

2 large eggs, soft or hard-boiled, and peeled

1 teaspoon olive oil

6 ounces Jones Canadian Bacon, julienned

1 small bunch of asparagus, cooked

5 ounces arugula, washed and dried

Directions

1. To make the salad dressing, put all the ingredients in a small jar with a tight-fitting lid. Shake the mixture until the contents have emulsified.

2. To make the salad, simply toss the dressing, asparagus, and salad greens together.

3. Put each half of the mixture on a different serving plate.

4. Now, into a skillet and over medium heat, sauté the bacon until lightly browned. Put on the salad along with the sliced avocado.

5. Garnish the breakfast salad with crispy shallots.

ZUCCHINI SALAD

Serves 4

Prep time: 20 minutes

Total Time: 20 minutes

Nutritional Information Per Serving: Calories 79, Carbs 4.5 g, Protein 5.5g, Fat 3g

Ingredients

2 tablespoons Italian dressing

1/3 cup red onion, finely chopped

1/2 cup feta cheese, crumbled

1 cup cherry tomatoes, halved

2 large zucchini, ends removed

Directions

1. Peel the zucchini lengthwise using a vegetable peeler into thin strips.

2. Rotate the zucchini after each strip to have a width that resembles a fettuccine.

3. Add the zucchini to a bowl along with the rest of the ingredients. Gently toss everything until blended.

4. *Cover and put in the refrigerator until ready to serve.*

EGG SALAD

Serves 1

Total time: 5 minutes

Nutritional Information Per Serving: Calories 415, Fat 38g, Protein 13g, Carbs 5g

Ingredients

¼ teaspoon black pepper

½ teaspoon pink Himalayan salt

1/8 medium white onion, chopped

2 celery stalks, chopped

1 teaspoon curry powder

2 ½ tablespoon mayonnaise

2 large eggs

Directions

1. Chop the eggs into chunks into a bowl.

2. Add the celery, onions, salt, pepper, curry, mayonnaise, and mix using a spoon.

3. You can serve immediately or refrigerate until ready to eat.

MAIN MEALS

CHICKEN LOMBARDY

Serves 6

Prep Time: 10 minutes

Cook Time: 45 minutes

Total Time: 55 minutes

Nutritional Information Per Serving: Calories 375, Carbs 4g, Protein 43g, Fat 20g

Ingredients

1 teaspoon Italian seasoning

1/2 cup Parmesan grated

1 1/2 cups grated mozzarella cheese

1/8 teaspoon xanthan gum

1/2 teaspoon pepper

1/2 teaspoon salt

1/4 cup heavy whipping cream

1 1/2 cups chicken broth

4 tablespoons butter, divided

8 oz sliced mushrooms

2 garlic cloves minced

1/2 small onion

2 pounds boneless skinless chicken breasts thin cut

Directions

1. Preheat your oven to 400 degrees F. Meanwhile, grease a 9 by 13-inch casserole dish.

2. Melt 2 tablespoons of butter in a large cast-iron skillet.

3. Once hot, sauté the onions, garlic, and mushrooms until the mushrooms are tender and the onions are translucent. This would take you about 10 minutes or so.

4. Remove the mushroom mixture from the skillet and set it aside. Now melt another 3 tablespoons of butter in the skillet, sear the chicken breasts until well browned, approximately 3 to 4 minutes on each side.

5. After each piece is brown, remove it from the skillet and put it in the casserole dish, but leave all the drippings in the skillet.

6. As soon as all the chicken is fully browned, add the garlic and mushroom mixture back in the skillet together with heavy whipping cream, chicken broth, and some salt and pepper.

7. Cook the mixture on medium-high heat for approximately 5 minutes while stirring and scraping the bottom of the skillet.

8. Turn off the stove, sprinkle 1/8 teaspoon of xanthan gum on top, and let the sauce thicken for about 4 to 10 minutes. You can also skip the xanthan gum if you like!

9. Once the sauce is thick to your liking, spoon it over the chicken, followed by the Parmesan cheese, and top with the mozzarella cheese.

10. Top the dish with a teaspoon of Italian seasoning and then bake Chicken Lombardy in the preheated oven at 450 degrees for about 12 to 14 minutes.

11. You can move the casserole dish to the top rack and then

set the oven to the broil setting to help brown the cheese.

12. Enjoy!

KETO LASAGNA

Served 6

Prep Time: 15 minutes

Cook Time: 40 minutes

Total Time: 55 minutes

Nutritional Information Per Serving: Calories 407, Carbs 4.1g, Protein 42.9g, Fat 23.9g

Ingredients

1 1/5 cups shredded cheese

4 Folios zero carb tortillas

1.5 pounds ground beef or turkey

1 cup Rao's marinara sauce

1/2 teaspoon garlic powder

3 tablespoons parsley

1 cup ricotta cheese whole milk

2 eggs

Directions

1. First, brown the ground turkey or beef in a skillet. Season the browned meat with some salt and pepper.

2. Mix 3 tablespoons parsley, 1 cup ricotta, 1/2 teaspoon garlic powder, and 2 eggs in a small bowl until well blended.

3. Spray the bottom of a medium-size casserole dish with non-stick spray or cooking oil.

4. Layer the bottom of the coated casserole dish with the zero-carb tortilla to make a crust at the bottom of the lasagna.

5. Add 1/4 of the ricotta cheese mixture to the tortilla and top with a thick layer of cooked ground meat.

6. Add approximately 1/4 cup of the marinara sauce to complete the first layer.

7. Repeat steps 5 and 6 for another three rounds to make the lasagna.

8. Finally, top the lasagna with some shredded cheese and enjoy!

CHEESY CHICKEN SKILLET

Serves 4

Prep Time: 35 minutes

Cook Time: 5 minutes

Total Time: 40 minutes

Nutritional Information Per Serving: Calories 295, Carbs 5g, Protein 22g, Fat 20g

Ingredients

1/2 cup Monterrey jack cheese

1 1/2 cups cheddar cheese

3/4 cup chicken broth or beef broth

2 tablespoons taco seasoning packet

1 12 oz. bag steamed riced cauliflower

1 can Rotel tomatoes

2 cups cooked shredded chicken or ground beef

3 garlic cloves minced

1/3 cup diced green pepper

1/3 cup diced onion

1 tablespoon butter

Directions

1. Melt butter in a cast iron and then sauté garlic, pepper,

and onion until softened.

2. Now add in the chicken broth, Rotel tomatoes, cauliflower, and the taco seasoning and stir to mix.

3. Cook the mixture on a medium heat setting until any excess liquid is absorbed or for about 10 minutes.

4. Now, add in the shredded chicken and stir to blend. In case you find the mixture too thick, add in extra chicken or beef broth.

5. Simmer the contents for approximately 5 minutes while covered.

6. Sprinkle some cheddar cheese on top, cover, and simmer the contents until the cheese has fully melted.

7. You can serve with jalapenos, cilantro, and sour cream if you like.

KETO BEEF STIR FRY

Serves 4

Prep Time: 10 minutes

Cook Time: 10 minutes

Total Time: 20 minutes

Nutritional Information Per Serving: Calories 314, Carbs 4.7g, Protein 23.5g, Fat 22.2g

Ingredients

3-inch scallion green part

3-inch scallion white part

2 red chili peppers thin slices

Ginger 3 inch long thin slices

3 tablespoons garlic minced

2 tablespoons toasted sesame oil

1 tablespoon fish sauce

2 tablespoons coconut aminos

Olive oil

1 pound beef tips thin sliced

Directions

1. In a bowl, whisk together sesame oil, fish sauce, and coconut aminos. Then drizzle the mixture on the beef tips and marinate the meat for approximately 15 to 30 minutes.

2. Add some oil into a large skillet, cook the beef tips for about 3 minutes until no longer pink.

3. Remove the beef from the skillet and set it aside.

4. Add in white scallion pieces, garlic, chili peppers, and ginger in the same pan.

5. Add in green scallion pieces and beef and toss until well combined. Serve and enjoy.

CHICKEN BROCCOLI CASSEROLE

Serves 8

Prep Time: 10 minutes

Cook Time: 35 minutes

Total Time: 45 minutes

Nutritional Information Per Serving: Calories 335, Carbs 7g, Protein 24g, Fat 22g

Ingredients

1/2 cup Parmesan cheese

1 pound broccoli florets

1 cup chicken bone broth

1/3 cup sour cream

8 ounces cream cheese

1/2 cup white cooking wine

6.5 ounces can mushroom, sliced

1/2 teaspoon tarragon

Salt and pepper to taste

1 tablespoon dried minced onion

3 cloves garlic

2 tablespoons butter

2 tablespoons olive oil

1 1/2 pounds boneless chicken breast

Directions

1. Begin by slicing the chicken into bite-sized chunks and then cooking the butter, olive oil, onion, and garlic.

2. As soon as the chicken is no longer pink, add in the rest of the ingredients.

3. Cook over medium heat, making sure that you stir for about about 10 minutes.

4. Pour the contents into a 9 by 13-inch casserole dish and top with some Parmesan cheese.

5. *Bake in the oven at 350 degrees for approximately 20 to 25 minutes.*

CHEESE STUFFED BACON CHEESEBURGER

Serves 2

Total Time: 25 minutes

Nutritional Information Per Serving: Calories 613.5, Carbs 1.5g, Protein 33g, Fat 51g

Ingredients

1 tablespoon butter

1 teaspoon Cajun seasoning

1/2 teaspoon pepper

1 teaspoon salt

2 oz. cheddar cheese

1 oz. mozzarella cheese

2 slices bacon, pre-cooked

8 ounces ground beef

Directions

1. Using all the spices, season the ground beef and mix lightly.

2. Cube the mozzarella cheese and slice the cheddar.

3. Using seasoned ground beef, make some patties. Once done, put the mozzarella inside and enclose the cheese with the meat.

4. In a pan, heat a tablespoon of butter until bubbling and hot.

Add one burger to the hot pan.

5. Cover using a cloche and cook for 2-3 minutes.

6. Then flip the burger and put the cheddar on top. Cover the pan with cloche again and cook for 1-2 minutes.

7. Finally, chop the bacon slice in half and put it over the burger. Serve.

INSTANT POT TURKEY BREAST

Serves 1 tenderloin

Prep Time: 5 minutes

Cook Time: 10 minutes

Total Time: 15 minutes

Nutritional Information Per Serving: Calories 376, Carbs 3g, Protein 79g, Fat 5g

Ingredients

1/4 teaspoon pepper

1 teaspoon salt

1/4 teaspoon sage

1/4 teaspoon thyme

1/2 teaspoon rosemary

1 teaspoon garlic powder

2 12 ounces each turkey breast tenderloins

1 cup broth or water

Directions

1. Put the rack into your instant pot or instead poach the turkey directly in the water.

2. Rub the spices and the herbs onto the meat, and then put

the turkey into the instant pot.

3. Lock the lid in place, press on the "Poultry" setting, and adjust cooking time to a range of 7 to 10 minutes, depending on the size of the turkey fillets.

4. As soon as cooking is done, quickly release the pressure and open the lid. Remove the cooked turkey breast.

5. You can serve the liquid from the cooking pan with the meat or save it as broth for another recipe.

CURRIED CAULIFLOWER WITH SHRIMP

Serves 4

Prep Time: 5 minutes

Cook Time: 15 minutes

Total Time: 20 minutes

Nutritional Information Per Serving: Calories 183, Carbs 8g, Protein 26g, Fat 4g

Ingredients

2 teaspoons extra virgin olive oil

Juice from half a lime

1 teaspoon smoked paprika

1 teaspoon cumin

2 teaspoons curry powder

3/4 cup low-sodium chicken stock

2 tablespoons parsley chopped

1 lb uncooked shrimp, peeled and deveined

2 cloves garlic, minced

1/2 red pepper chopped

1 onion chopped

1 bag green giant riced cauliflower frozen

Salt + pepper to taste

Directions

1. In a skillet, over medium heat, add some olive oil and heat until hot.

2. Add in chopped red pepper and onions, and then season with pepper and salt.

3. Cook the mixture until soft, or for approximately 3 or 4 minutes.

4. Add in the 2 cloves of garlic and cook for another 1 minute or so.

5. Add all the riced cauliflower into the skillet and mix using a wooden spoon.

6. Now add in smoked paprika, curry, and cumin and stir to mix.

7. Then add in the chicken broth and reduce the heat to medium-low.

8. Season the uncooked shrimp with salt and pepper, and then nestle them over the riced cauliflower.

9. Cook until the shrimp cooks through, or for approximately 2 to 3 minutes.

10. Uncover the shrimp and add in some parsley. Also, squeeze in some lime juice and stir.

11. Taste and adjust the seasoning as required, and then remove it from heat and serve.

STUFFED SALMON ROLLS

Serves 4

Prep Time: 15 minutes

Cook Time: 20 minutes

Total Time: 35 minutes

Nutritional Information Per Serving: Calories 400, Carbs 8.8g, Protein 43.8g, Fat 21.7g

Ingredients

2 tablespoons lemon juice

1/2 cup chicken broth

1 tablespoon butter

1/2 pound asparagus, trimmed

Salt and pepper to taste

2 teaspoons lemon zest

2 tablespoons basil, chopped

1/2 cup Parmesan cheese, grated

1 (12 ounces) container ricotta

4 (5 ounces) salmon fillets, skins removed

2 tablespoons lemon juice

Directions

1. Season the salmon with pepper and salt, and then lay them

with the skin side facing up.

2. Top the salmon fillets with lemon zest, basil, Parmesan, ricotta, salt, and pepper. Add a few spears of asparagus, and roll the mixture up.

3. Put the mixture on a greased baking sheet with the seam side facing down and bake in a preheated oven at 425 degrees F for about 15 to 20 minutes or until the salmon is cooked.

4. Over medium heat, melt some butter in a saucepan and then add the lemon juice and broth.

5. Heat for 3 to 5 minutes.

6. Serve the rolls with lemon sauce and garnish with lemon zest and basil.

CHEESY TUNA SPINACH CASSEROLE

Serves 4

Prep Time: 5 minutes

Cook Time: 30 minutes

Total Time: 35 minutes

Nutritional Information Per Serving: Calories 638, Carbs 6g, Protein 38g, Fat 52g

Ingredients

4 slices provolone or mozzarella cheese

9 ounces frozen spinach, drained

10 ounces canned tuna

1 tablespoon dried parsley

1 ½ cups Parmesan cheese

1/2 cup unsweetened almond milk

1 cup heavy cream

1 clove garlic, minced

1/4 cup butter

Directions

1. In a medium saucepan, over medium-low heat, add some butter and melt. Once melted, add in garlic.

2. As soon as the garlic is golden in color, add almond milk and cream.

3. Stir the mixture for approximately 4 minutes or so, and then whisk in Parmesan.

4. Now stir in spinach, tuna, and parsley, and then cook over medium heat while stirring now and again until bubbly.

5. Spoon the mixture into a lightly greased casserole dish and top with sliced cheese if you like.

6. Bake in the oven at 375 degrees F until bubbly or for approximately 20 minutes.

DESSERTS

BERRIES WITH CHOCOLATE GANACHE

Serves 6

Prep Time: 10 minutes

Cook Time: 5 minutes

Total Time: 15 minutes

Nutritional Information Per Serving: Calories 286.3, Carbs 8.1g, Protein 4g, Fat 17.6g

Ingredients

8 ounces strawberries

1/2 teaspoons vanilla extract

2 cups red raspberries

8-ounce chocolate chips, sugar-free

2 cups fresh blueberries

1/3 cup heavy cream

Directions

1. Mix the fruits and put them in dessert bowls.

2. Heat the heavy cream and chocolate chips over low heat until melted, or microwave the mixture for around 30 seconds.

3. Add in the vanilla and stir to get a smooth consistency.

4. Cool slightly and then serve.

FUDGE BOMBS

Yields 12

Prep Time: 15 minutes

Cook Time: 3 hours 15 minutes

Total Time: 3 hours 30 minutes

Nutritional Information Per Serving: Calories 163, Carbs 3.86g, Protein 1.0g, Fat 16.18g

Ingredients

3 ounces of 70% dark chocolate pieces

1 teaspoon of vanilla

3 ounces of butter (at room temperature)

2 cups of heavy whipping cream

Directions

1. In a heavy saucepan, boil the heavy cream for about 1 minute while stirring continuously.

2. Lower the heat to simmer until the cream has reduced in half or simmer for approximately 20 minutes.

3. Add in butter, let it melt, and then remove the contents from heat. Add in chocolate along with preferred flavors and keep stirring until chocolate pieces have melted.

4. Now, pour the mixture into a baking dish, 7 by 7 inches. Let the contents cool in the fridge for around 3 hours or so.

5. Cut into pieces and top with some cocoa powder. Keep any remaining fudge chilled or frozen.

ALMOND FUDGE BROWNIES

Yields 16

Prep Time: 5 minutes

Cook Time: 11 minutes

Total Time: 16 minutes

Nutritional Information Per Serving: Calories 118, Carbs 5g, Protein 5g, Fat 11g

Ingredients

1/2 teaspoon baking powder

10 tablespoon cocoa powder, unsweetened

3 large eggs

1/2 cup Swerve Confectioners or 3/4 cup powdered erythritol

1 cup almond butter

Directions

1. Blend erythritol and almond butter in a food processor.

2. Add in baking powder, cocoa powder, and eggs. Then season with some salt.

3. Transfer the batter to a greased baking pan and smooth the mixture with a spatula.

4. Bake for approximately 11 minutes at 325 degrees F. Cool fully

to allow it to firm up and then serve.

COCONUT LEMON BARS

Yields 12

Prep Time: 15 minutes

Cook Time: 2 hours 15 minutes

Total Time: 2 hours 30 minutes

Nutritional Information: Calories 64, Carbs 2.5g, Protein 0.44g, Fat 6.1g

Ingredients

¾ cup of splenda or stevia

1/3 cup of coconut oil

2 tablespoons of fresh lemon rind

3 cups of shredded coconut, unsweetened

Directions

1. Line a casserole dish using parchment paper and set it aside. Meanwhile, mix all the ingredients in a large bowl until well-mixed.

2. Pour the batter into the casserole dish and gently press it into place.

3. Store in the freezer for a minimum of 2 hours, or preferably overnight.

4. Cut the dessert into squares using a knife and serve. Store any remaining bars frozen in a freezer.

PEANUT BUTTER COOKIES

Yields 15

Prep Time: 15 minutes

Cook Time: 10 minutes

Total Time: 25 minutes

Nutritional Information Per Serving: Calories 110, Carbs 3g, Protein 5g, Fat 9g

Ingredients

1/2 cup Swerve, Granular

1 large egg

1 cup crunchy peanut butter

Directions

1. Preheat the oven to 350 degrees F. Meanwhile, line a cookie sheet using parchment paper.

2. In a mixing bowl, mix all the ingredients until well incorporated.

3. Make 15 one-inch balls using your hands or a cookie scoop and put them on the parchment-lined cookie sheet. Press on them using a fork to make a crisscross pattern.

4. Bake until the tops are golden brown, or for about 10 to 13 minutes. Then allow the cookies to cool before serving.

PEANUT BUTTER DROPS

Yields 20

Prep Time: 10 minutes

Cook Time: 10 minutes

Total Time: 20 minutes

Nutritional Information Per Serving: Calories 64, Carbs 4.33g, Protein 3.25g, Fat 4.10g

Ingredients

6 servings of 1 packet Splenda

1 large egg

8 ounces peanut butter

Directions

1. Mix all the ingredients to have a firm dough.

2. Roll the dough into tiny drops and place them on an ungreased cookie sheet.

3. Bake in the preheated oven at 350 degrees F for approximately 9 to 10 minutes.

4. Serve and enjoy.

FRUITY CHEESECAKE MOUSSE

Serves 8

Prep Time: 15 minutes

Total Time: 3 hours 15 minutes

Nutritional Information Per Serving: Calories 201, Carb: 4.5g, Protein 3.3g, Fat 19.9g

Ingredients

1 tablespoon sour cream

1/2 cup boiling water

4 packets sugar-free gelatin

1 cup heavy cream

1 cup cream cheese

Directions

1. First, boil half a cup of water and then melt the unsweetened gelatin in the boiling water, stirring, until fully dissolved.

2. Beat the cream cheese until you get a smooth consistency, and then stir in the dissolved gelatin.

3. In a bowl, whip the heavy cream until peaks form, and then fold in the cream cheese and gelatin mixture.

4. Now stir in sour cream and keep the mixture frozen for ap-

proximately 3 hours.

KETO BROWNIE

Yields 12

Total Time: 45 minutes

Nutritional Information Per Serving: Calories 178, Carbs 3.5g, Protein 4.5g, Fat 17g

Ingredients

4.2 ounces cream cheese, softened

3 - 5 tablespoons granulated sweetener

2 teaspoons vanilla

1/2 teaspoon baking powder

2.2 ounces unsweetened cocoa

5.6 ounces melted butter

6 eggs

Directions

1. Put all the ingredients in a mixing bowl, and blend until smooth using a stick blender with a blade attachment.

2. Pour the batter into a 21 by 8.5-inch baking dish. Bake at 350 degrees F until well cooked at the center. Brownies should Take 20-25 minutes.

3. Slice the brownie into squares, triangle wedges, or rectangle bars and serve.

KETO POPSICLES

Serves 6

Prep time: 5 minutes

Cook time: 5 minutes

Freezing time: 4 hours

Total time: 4 hours 10 minutes

Nutritional Information Per Serving: Calories 295, Fat 24.8g, Protein 3.5g, Carbs 4.9g

Ingredients

1 cup raspberries

1 teaspoon vanilla extract

¼ teaspoon sea salt

¼ cup powdered allulose

1 ¼ cups coconut cream

¾ cup sugar-free white chocolate chips

Directions

1. Place a double boiler on the stove and put the chocolate chips into the double boiler. Stir frequently until all the chocolate has melted.

2. Add in powdered allulose, sea salt, and coconut cream and whisk until dissolved.

3. Remove from heat, then stir in the vanilla.

4. Put three raspberries in 6 popsicle molds, then pour the cream mixture into the molds until they are halfway filled. Add 3 more raspberries, then fill with the cream mixture.

5. Put a popsicle stick into each mold and freeze for about 4 hours or until they are solid.

KETO FLAN

Serves 6

Prep time: 5 minutes

Cook time: 45 minutes

Cooling time: 1 hour

Total time: 50 minutes

Nutritional Information Per Serving: Calories 331, Fat 33.3g, Carbs 2.9g, Protein 4.8g

Ingredients

1 cup powdered monk fruit sweetener

2 teaspoons vanilla extract

1 pinch sea salt

2 cups heavy cream

6 egg yolks

¼ cup water

Directions

1. Preheat your oven to 350 degrees F.

2. In a pan over low heat, ½ cup of the sweetener with ¼ cup of water. Heat this until it dissolves.

3. Increase the heat, bring the mixture to a boil, and then simmer for about 20 minutes without stirring until you have a golden syrup.

4. Very quickly, divide the syrup among 6 (6-ounces ramekins) and tilt the ramekins in different directions to spread the syrup. Put the ramekins in a baking dish measuring 9x13.

5. Whisk the egg yolks in a medium bowl.

6. Heat the remaining sweetener, salt, and heavy cream in a pan over medium heat. Once bubbles begin to form around the edges, remove from the heat, add in the vanilla extract, and mix.

7. Pour the cream mixture slowly into the bowl with egg yolks as you whisk constantly. This is known as tampering and is what forms the custard.

8. Pour the custard into the ramekins through a fine-mesh sieve.

9. Pour some hot water into the baking dish, ensuring that you fill it up to halfway up the sides of the ramekins.

10. Bake for 20-30 minutes and ensure you rotate the pan halfway through until the flan sets but still jiggles a bit at the center.

11. Remove from the oven but let the ramekins sit in the water bath for about an hour to cool.

12. Dry the ramekins, cover them with some plastic wrap, and put them in the fridge overnight and can stay up to four days.

13. Run a knife along the edges of the ramekin until the flan starts to rotate inside the ramekin.

14. Place a plate on top of the ramekin, then invert and shake up a little bit to release the flan.

SOUPS AND SNACKS

ASPARAGUS AND LEEK SOUP

Serves 4

Prep Time: 15 minutes

Cook Time: 15 minutes

Total Time: 30 minutes

Nutritional Information Per Serving: Calories 167.7, Carbs 7.6g, Protein 4.9g, Fat 13.8g

Ingredients

1/3 cup heavy cream

1 14.5 ounces can chicken broth

1 teaspoon garlic

3/4 pound asparagus

1 cup leek, freshly chopped

2 tablespoons butter stick, unsalted

Directions

1. Into a large pot, over medium-high heat, melt butter and then add in the leeks. Sauté for about 3 minutes and then add in the asparagus— cook for a minute.

2. Add in the garlic and sauté for an additional 30 seconds.

3. Now, add broth into the pot and let it boil. Reduce the heat and

simmer for 8-10 minutes covered.

4. Once the asparagus is tender, mix in the pepper and salt and then blend the soup in a processor until smooth.

5. Return the soup to the cooking pot to heat through before you serve. You can season with ground pepper and salt if desired.

CHICKEN SOUP

Serves 6

Prep time: 10 minutes

Cook time: 22 minutes

Total time: 32 minutes

Nutritional Information Per Serving: Calories 196, Fat 10.4g, Carbs 5.8g, Protein 26.4g

Ingredients

2 cups riced cauliflower

1 pound cubed boneless, skinless chicken thighs

4 cups chicken broth

½ teaspoon paprika

½ teaspoon dried thyme leaves

2 garlic cloves, minced

Salt and pepper to taste

¼ cup chopped onions

2 celery stalks, chopped

2 tablespoons avocado oil

Directions

1. In a large pan over medium heat, heat the oil.

2. Add the onions and celery and season with pepper and salt.

Cook while stirring until tender, for about 5 minutes.

3. Add the thyme, garlic, and paprika and cook until fragrant. Add in the broth, stir and bring to a boil.

4. Add in the riced cauliflower and the chicken and reduce the heat to simmer. Cook until the chicken is cooked through. You can adjust the salt and pepper to your taste.

MUSHROOM SOUP

Serves 4

Prep time: 10 minutes

Cook time: 50 minutes

Total time: 1 hour

Total Nutritional Information Per Serving: Calories 215, Protein 5g, Fat 8g, Carbs 3g

Ingredients

1 cup heavy cream

4 egg yolks

2 cups water

7 ounces cream cheese

5 tablespoons dry white wine

¼ teaspoon ground black pepper

1 ½ teaspoons sea salt

1 tablespoon dried thyme

3 garlic cloves

1 pound mushrooms

4 ounces yellow onions

2 tablespoons butter

7 ounces parma ham

Directions

1. Preheat the oven to 300 degrees F.

2. Place parma ham slices on a baking sheet that has been lined with parchment paper and bake in the oven in the upper rack. Check on them every 5 minutes and flip a few times while drying. This will take about 30 minutes to crisp up.

3. Sauté garlic, mushrooms, and onions in butter in a pot over medium heat until it is golden, then season with pepper, salt, and thyme.

4. Add cheese, wine, and water and stir. Bring this to a boil and boil for a few minutes, lower the heat, and simmer for about 15 minutes.

5. Whisk the heavy cream until the soft peaks start to form, then add the yolks and mix.

6. Now, turn off the heat and fold the cream into the soup.

7. Serve the soup and put the parma ham on top.

BROCCOLI CHEESE SOUP

Serves 8

Total time: 20 minutes

Nutritional Information Per Serving: Calories 292, Fat 25g, Protein 13g, Carbs 4g

Ingredients

3 cups cheddar cheese

1 cup heavy cream

3 ½ cups chicken broth

4 garlic cloves, minced

4 cups broccoli, cut into florets

Directions

1. Sauté garlic for about a minute in a pot over medium heat.

2. Add the broccoli, cream, and broth and bring to a boil. Now lower the heat and simmer for about 20 minutes until the broccoli is tender, then turn off the heat.

3. Using a slotted spoon, remove about 1/3 of the broccoli pieces and put them aside.

4. Puree the remaining broccoli using an immersion blender.

5. Put on the heat to low, add the cheese ½ cup at a time while stirring and continue to do so until it has melted. Puree once more to ensure that it is smooth.

6. Remove from heat, add in the broccoli florets you had set aside, stir and serve.

BACON CHEESE BURGER SOUP

Serves: 10

Prep time: 20 minutes

Cook time: 60 minutes

Total time: 1 hour 20 minutes

Nutritional Information Per Serving: Calories 372, Protein 19.1g, Fat 30.9g, Carbs 3.6g

Ingredients

8 slices bacon, cooked and crumbled

1 cup heavy cream

1 ½ cups shredded cheddar cheese

4 garlic cloves, minced

1 onion, diced

1 ½ pounds ground beef

½ teaspoon black pepper

1 teaspoon sea salt

2 tablespoons chopped flat-leaf parsley

2 tablespoons Worcestershire sauce

2 tablespoons Dijon mustard

1/3 cup chopped dill pickles

1 tomato, diced

4 cups beef stock

Directions

1. Heat a Dutch oven over medium heat. Add the onions, garlic, and ground beef and cook until the ground beef is cooked through and has browned.

2. Add the Worcestershire sauce, Dijon mustard, pickles, tomato, beef stock, pepper, and salt and bring to a boil. Lower the heat to medium, then simmer for 30 minutes.

3. Add in the heavy cream and cheddar cheese, lower the heat to low, and simmer for about 30 minutes.

4. Add the bacon when serving.

KETO PIZZA CHIPS

Serves 2

Prep Time: 5 minutes

Cook Time: 10 minutes

Total Time: 15 minutes

Nutritional Information Per Serving: Calories 130, Carbs 2g, Protein 7g, Fat 10g

Ingredients

1 teaspoon Italian seasoning

1/4 cup shredded mozzarella cheese

1/8 cup fresh grated Parmesan

14 or 1-ounce pepperoni

Directions

1. Preheat your oven to 400 degrees F.

2. Meanwhile, remove any excess oil from the pepperoni and put it on a baking sheet lined with parchment paper or at the bottom of a muffin tin.

3. Sprinkle the pepperoni with grated Parmesan, mozzarella cheese, and a little Italian seasoning.

4. Bake the mixture for approximately 8 to 10 minutes.

5. Remove the pepperoni from the oven and let it cool and crisp up.

6. Using a towel, blot off any excess oils from both sides of the pepperoni.

7. You can now serve the pizza chips with ranch or marinara sauce if you like.

AVOCADO DEVILED EGGS

Serves 8

Total Time: 30 minutes

Nutritional Information Per Serving: Calories 213, Carbs 5.6g, Protein 10.9g, Fat 16.6g

Ingredients

1 lime, juiced and zested

1/4 cup mayonnaise

2 tablespoon cilantro, chopped

1 tablespoon chile powder

2 jalapeño peppers, seeded and finely chopped

1/2 teaspoon salt

1 tablespoon Dijon mustard

1 tablespoon capers, finely chopped

1 tablespoon ground cumin

1 ripe, fresh avocado, seeded and peeled

12 large eggs, hard-boiled and peeled

Directions

1. Begin by cutting the eggs in half lengthwise. Remove the yolks, then, using a spoon, mash the yolks thoroughly and then add in the avocado. Mash once more.

2. Combine the mashed avocado and yolks mixture with

jalapeno, salt, lime juice, mustard, lime zest, capers, cumin, and mayonnaise.

3. Fill the egg whites with the avocado and egg yolk mixture around one tablespoon in each half.

4. Season with the chile powder and serve garnished with cilantro if you like.

KETO PROTEIN BALLS

Yields 24 balls

Prep Time: 10 minutes

Total Time: 30 minutes

Nutritional Information Per Serving: Calories 92, Carbs 3g, Protein 4g, Fat 7.5g

Ingredients

2 teaspoons vanilla extract

1/2 cup powdered erythritol

1/2 cup protein powder

1/2 cup peanuts, optional

1 cup thick and creamy peanut butter, salted

Directions

1. Mix the protein powder, peanut butter, vanilla, and powdered erythritol in a food processor or blender until smooth.

2. Pulse the ingredients while scraping down the sides when required until you get a uniform creamy mixture that is dense and can be pressed together.

3. If you find the mixture too thin, add some extra protein powder and more powdered erythritol.

4. You can also stir in chopped peanuts if you like it somehow crunchy. Then pulse once or twice to mix the peanuts

in but do not blend them thoroughly as they'll release oil and change the consistency of your protein balls.

5. Keep the dough frozen for around 20 minutes to harden the mixture.

6. Get a spoon or a cookie scoop, scoop dough balls, and then roll the dough into balls using wet hands.

7. Store the peanut butter protein balls in the fridge until ready to serve.

PARMESAN ZUCCHINI FRIES

Prep Time: 10 minutes

Cook Time: 20 minutes

Total Time: 30 minutes

Serves 4

Nutritional Information Per Serving: Calories 213, Carbs 4g, Protein 21g, Fat 15g

Ingredients

1/4 teaspoon garlic powder

1 large egg

3/4 cup grated Parmesan cheese

2 medium zucchini

1/4 tsp black pepper, optional

Directions

1. Preheat your oven to 425 degrees F, and then line your baking sheet with foil or parchment paper. Lightly grease the baking sheet.

2. Cut individual zucchini in half lengthwise a couple of times until you have eight long sticks from each squash.

3. Cut the eight sticks crosswise to get 16 bars that measure

about 10 centimeters or 4 inches long. In case the zucchini sticks appear wet, pat them dry with a paper towel.

4. Set up two shallow bowls, one with the grated cheese, black pepper, and garlic mixture and the other with 1 beaten egg.

5. Dip individual squash stick in the egg, shake off any excess egg, and press into the Parmesan and garlic mixture to coat all the sides. You can use one of your hands in the egg and the other for the cheese mixture.

6. Put the squash on the lined baking sheet in a single layer making sure the sticks do not touch.

7. Bake in the preheated oven for approximately 20 minutes. Make sure that you rotate the pan and flip the fries while halfway through.

8. Put the dish under the broiler and broil until dark golden and crispy, or for approximately 2 to 3 minutes.

ROASTED PECANS

Serves 8

Prep Time: 5 minutes

Cook Time: 12 minutes

Total Time: 17 minutes

Nutritional Information Per Serving: Calories 213, Carbs 4.7g, Protein 2.38g, Fat 22.3g

Ingredients

2 tablespoons confectioners' erythritol

2 tablespoons Pumpkin Pie Spice

1 teaspoon pure vanilla extract

3 tablespoons salted butter, melted

2 cups raw pecan

Directions

1. Preheat the oven to 350 degrees F. Meanwhile, use parchment paper to line a rimmed baking sheet.

2. In a mixing bowl, combine pecans, vanilla, and butter. Toss the nuts with a rubber spatula to coat with the melted butter.

3. Evenly distribute the pumpkin spice and sweetener over the mixture and toss to coat well with the raw pecans.

4. Spread the coated pecans across the lined baking sheet in a single layer and bake for approximately 12 minutes.

SMOOTHIES AND ALCOHOLIC DRINKS

CUCUMBER SPINACH SMOOTHIE

Serves 1

Total Time: 15 minutes

Nutritional Information Per Serving: Calories 330, Carbs 5g, Protein 10g, Fats 32g

Ingredients

1-2 tablespoons MCT oil

1/4 teaspoon xanthan gum

12 drops liquid stevia

1 cup coconut milk

7 ice cubes

2.5 ounces cucumber, peeled and cubed

2 handfuls spinach

Directions

1. Toss 2 handfuls of spinach into a blender, then add in MCT oil, xanthan gum, stevia, coconut milk, and the ice cubes.

2. Peel the cucumber, cube it and place it over the top. Now blend the ingredients for around 1-2 minutes to incorporate them.

3. Finally, pour the smoothie into a glass and serve.

STRAWBERRY SMOOTHIE

Serves: 4

Total time: 5 minutes

Nutritional Information Per Serving: Calories 40, Carbs 2g, Protein 1g, Fat 1g

Ingredients

1 cup frozen strawberries

2 cups crushed ice

½ cup Greek yogurt

1 cup almond milk

Directions

1. Add the milk, yogurt, and ice into the blender and process.

2. Now add in the strawberries and blend until smooth.

KETO GREEN SMOOTHIE

Serves 2

Total time: 5 minutes

Nutritional Information Per Serving: Calories 141, Protein 4g, Carbs 4.8g, Fat 10.8g

Ingredients

2 tablespoons lemon juice

1 tablespoon peanut butter

1 cup unsweetened almond milk

2 ounces cucumber

1 celery stick, chopped

½ avocado, peeled

1-ounce kale leaves

Directions

1. Add all the ingredients into your blender and blend until smooth. You can serve it immediately or store it in the fridge to have later.

PEANUT BUTTER SMOOTHIE

Serves 2

Total time: 5 minutes

Nutritional Information Per Serving: Calories 172, Protein 5.2g, Fat 15.4g, Carbs 4.7g

Ingredients

1 tablespoon unsweetened cocoa powder

1 cup crushed ice

¼ cup heavy cream

3 tablespoons monk fruit

2 tablespoons peanut butter

1 cup unsweetened almond milk

Directions

1. Blend all the ingredients until smooth.

KETO PROTEIN SMOOTHIE

Serves 1

Total time: 2 minutes

Nutritional Information Per Serving: Calories 538, Protein 28g, Fat 39g, Carbs 6g

Ingredients

1 tablespoon chia seeds

½ teaspoon ginger

2 teaspoon vanilla extract

½ tablespoon coconut oil

1 scoop protein powder

1 cup unsweetened coconut milk

2 tablespoons cacao butter

2 tablespoons monk fruit sweetener

5 ice cubes

Directions

1. Add the milk first into the blender, then add the rest of the ingredients and process until smooth.

KETO MARGARITA

Serves 1

Total time: 5 minutes

Nutritional Information Per Serving: Calories 104, Carbs 3g,

Ingredients

1/4 cup water

1 tablespoon allulose

2 tablespoons lime juice

Ice

Directions

1. Put all the ingredients in a blender or cocktail shaker and puree or shake until slushy.

2. Pour over ice into a glass and enjoy.

VODKA MOJITO

Serves 1

Total time: 5 minutes

Nutritional Information: Calories 109, Carbs 2g

Ingredients

1 shot vodka

2g granulated stevia

2 tablespoons lime juice

4 fresh mint leaves

1 splash club soda

Slices of lime for garnish

Directions

1. Smash the mint leaves with lime and stevia using a muddler and put this in a glass.

2. Add vodka and club soda into the glass.

3. Add some ice and garnish with a slice of lime and mint.

WHISKEY SMASH

Serves 1

Total time: 2 minutes

Nutritional Information: Calories 214, Fat 1g, Protein 1 g, Carbs 0.5g

Ingredients

2 ounces whiskey

2 drops of stevia

¼ lime

8 mint leaves plus more for garnishing

Crushed ice

Directions

1. Place the stevia, lime wedges, and mint leaves in a mason jar, then mash using a muddle to release the juice.

2. Add whiskey and some ice, cover, and shake for about 30 seconds.

3. Pour into a glass, add more ice and garnish with mint.

KETO EGGNOG

Serves 6

Prep time: 5 minutes

Cook time: 10 minutes

Chill time: 3 hours

Total time: 3 hours 15 minutes

Nutritional Information Per Serving: Calories 271, Fat 26.9g, Protein 4.6g, Carbs 2.5g

Ingredients

1 teaspoon vanilla extract

1 cup bourbon

½ teaspoon cinnamon

½ teaspoon nutmeg

1 ½ cups heavy cream

1 ½ cups unsweetened almond milk

½ cup sweetener

6 egg yolks

Directions

1. Beat the yolks using a hand mixer until light yellow. Add in the sweetener little by little as you beat until dissolved, then set aside.

2. Mix the almond milk, nutmeg, cinnamon, and cream in a pan.

Bring this to a boil while stirring occasionally. Once it starts to boil, remove it from heat.

3. As you constantly whisk, pour the hot mixture into the bowl with the yolks in a thin stream.

4. Pour the resulting mixture back into the pan, then heat over medium heat while constantly whisking until the mixture begins to thicken slightly. Make sure that you do not boil.

5. Add the bourbon now, pour the eggnog into a bowl, cover, and put it in the fridge for about 3-4 hours.

6. Serve with some whipped cream that is sugar-free.

MIXED BERRY MOJITO

Serves 2

Total time: 5 minutes

Nutritional Information Per Serving: Calories 159, Fat 0.3g, Protein 0.9g, Carbs 4.7g

Ingredients

1 cup sparkling water

½ cup white rum

2 tablespoons powdered erythritol

4 tablespoons lime juice

½ cup mint

½ cup raspberries and blackberries

Ice cubes

Directions

1. Place the berries, powdered erythritol, lime juice, and mint in a glass.

2. Use a long spoon to crush the berries to release flavor.

3. Pour in the white rum, and then add in the sparkling water.

4. Garnish with more mint leaves and berries and enjoy.

MEAL PLANNING TIPS

When meal planning, it's advisable to plan several meals ahead of time along with a grocery list that should help you buy the foods you need.

When making a grocery list, first decide the recipes you want to complete in advance, then pick those with similar ingredients to help simplify the grocery list and avoid unnecessary surplus.

Also, consider various plant proteins, veggies, and sauces that can effortlessly mix and match. If you shop with pay-by-weight bulk bins, be free to buy as much of the supplies as you need. You may consider doubling ingredients for your favorite recipes.

From the recipes included in this book, here is the suggested grocery list to get you started:

KETO RECIPES
SHOPPING LIST

KETO RECIPES SHOPPING LIST

Meat and Fish

2 1/2 pounds chicken breasts, skinless and boneless

1 1/2 pounds sausage meat, gluten-free

12 ounces pork Sausage Roll

1 can of sardines in olive oil or brine

1 ½ pound ground turkey

24 ounces ground beef

9 ounces Canadian bacon

1 pound uncooked shrimp

140g Tinned tuna

1 pound Beef tips

4 (5 ounces) Salmon fillets, skins removed

2 (12 ounces) turkey breast tenderloin

8 ounces pepperoni

DAIRY, PLANT MILK AND EGGS

16 fl. ounces almond milk, unsweetened

8 fl. ounces coconut milk, unsweetened

4 ounces Monterrey jack cheese

96 pastured eggs

20 fl. ounces heavy whipping cream

8 ounces ricotta cheese whole milk

6 ounces Lemon yogurt

8 fl. ounces of buttermilk

4 fl. Ounces sour cream

12 ounces mozzarella cheese

4 slices provolone cheese

4 ounces feta cheese

30.2 ounces Cream cheese

4 Duck eggs

12 ounces hard goat cheese, grated

8 fl. ounces milk

8 ounces pepper jack cheese

VEGGIES

2 pounds broccoli florets

9 ounces frozen spinach

4 1/2 pounds fresh spinach

2 red onions

1 bag riced cauliflower or cauli-rice

1/2 cup fresh basil sprigs

2 tablespoons basil, chopped

2.5 ounces cucumber

200g Swiss chard or dark-leaf kale

1/4 pound salad greens

1 medium spring onion or a bunch of chives

1 small head of lettuce

2 1/4 pounds medium asparagus, cut into thirds

1 small bunch of asparagus

1 (14-ounce) canned artichoke hearts

10 ounces mushrooms

4 large zucchini, ends removed

8 ounces cherry tomatoes

2 medium tomatoes

1 can Rotel tomatoes

1 large green pepper

3 inch Scallion

2 Red chili peppers

Ginger, 3 inches long

24 ounces shredded coconut, unsweetened

1 leek

7 Garlic cloves

A bunch of cilantro

2 jalapeño peppers

FRUITS

10 lemons

3 limes

10 ounces strawberries

1 pound red raspberries

1 pound fresh blueberries

2 Fresh avocados

FATS AND OILS

2 ounces mayonnaise

4 fl. Ounces avocado oil

10 fl. Ounces olive oil

20g ghee or lard

1 tablespoon Flaxseed oil

10 ounces butter

2 tablespoons toasted sesame oil

8 ounces almond butter

16 ounces peanut butter

14.5 ounce can of organic coconut cream

1-2 tablespoons MCT Oil

FLOURS

8 ounces golden flaxseed or flax meal

2 ounces coconut flour

1 tablespoon whole psyllium husks

4 Folios zero carb tortillas

NUTS AND SEEDS

8 ounces walnuts

1 pound raw almonds

½ cup Flaked almonds, toasted

2 cups Raw pecan

BROTHS AND COOKING LIQUIDS

6 fl. Ounces low sodium chicken stock

1 1/2 teaspoons Red wine vinegar

6 fl. Ounces chicken broth or beef broth

4 fl. Ounces white cooking wine

1/3 cup Apple cider vinegar

6 cups Filtered water

SPICES, CONDIMENTS, AND OTHERS

12 fresh mint leaves

Black pepper, as per your taste

Sea salt, as required

Kosher salt

Pink Himalayan salt

White pepper

Dried oregano

Splenda

8 ounces chocolate chips, sugar-free

1 Taco seasoning packet

1 teaspoon Celery seed

4 ounces Swerve confectioners

2 teaspoons Xanthan gum

Cocoa powder, unsweetened

1 teaspoon Sage

Keto hollandaise sauce

8 ounces Rao's marinara sauce

Parsley

Minced onion flakes

Baking soda

Anchovy paste

Smoked paprika

Curry powder

Dijon mustard

Worcestershire sauce

Cinnamon

Vanilla extract

Vanilla stevia

Maple extract

8 ounces salsa

Chili powder

Cumin

Coriander

Dill

Chervil

Italian dressing

Italian seasoning

Tarragon

Erythritol

Fish sauce

Coconut aminos

Cajun seasoning

4 packets sugar-free gelatin

Dried dill weed

VEE LEWIS

Chile powder

Keto-protein vanilla

Pumpkin pie spice

Club soda

Sparkling water

ALCOHOLIC DRINKS

1 shot vodka

2 ounces whiskey

8 fl. Ounces bourbon

4 fl. Ounces white rum

2 fl. Ounces tequila

OTHER WAYS TO FIGHT OBESITY

As mentioned earlier in a previous chapter, while your diet contributes significantly to being obese, other things also come into play, such as physical activity levels, stress, and sleep. We have already addressed the diet part by adopting the ketogenic diet. Let us now look at how you can fight obesity while addressing other causes of obesity.

EXERCISE

According to various national and international guidelines, it's recommended that you get a minimum of 150 minutes of moderate pace physical activity in a week. This translates to approximately 30 minutes of exercise in a day for about five days a week. If you find hitting the gym harder, a 2015 study shows that brisk walking at a fast pace can help promote weight loss. Also, try having an active day by walking to the office, taking regular stretch breaks, and other workout routines. In addition, research shows that having a pet, particularly a dog, can help you exercise more through normal walking.

HAVE ADEQUATE SLEEP

Research shows that late sleeping right from adolescence to adult age can directly contribute to increased BMI over time. A related study reveals that late bedtime, equivalent to fewer sleep hours, increases obesity, particularly for 4 to 5-year-old kids. Getting less than 9.5 hours of night sleep made it more likely for children to develop obesity with time. For adults, the CDC recommends that you get a minimum of 7 hours of sleep a day.

LEARN TO RELAX

Chronic stress typically increases cortisol level, a stress hormone that is linked to weight gain. Anxiety and depression can also lead to poor food choices, cravings and make it harder for you to exercise. Therefore, it is paramount to find ways to relax and calm down when stressed. There are various ways of relaxing and fighting stress, such as meditation, going for a walk, doing yoga, listening to music, and chatting with friends.

Conclusion

It's my sincere hope the book has been of much help to you. It's now time to put into practice what you've already learned, and in no time, you're highly likely to succeed with the diet. Get out and begin your Ketogenic lifestyle for ultimate transformation to your ideal body weight.

Good luck!

www.ingramcontent.com/pod-product-compliance
Lightning Source LLC
Chambersburg PA
CBHW061346250726
48657CB00004B/1348